ADJUSTING TO LIFE WITH DIABETES + COMPLICATIONS

Dr. Susan Guzman
Dr. Dennis Gooler

I0439492

Created by

Dynamic Diabetes Solutions
San Diego, California
2014

Copyright, authors and disclaimer

E-Booklet Title	Adjusting to Life with Diabetes + Complications
Primary author	Dr. Susan J. Guzman
Contributing author	Dr. Dennis D. Gooler
Copyright	Copyright @ 2014. All rights reserved.
Publisher	Dynamic Diabetes Solutions
Contact	Dr. Dennis Gooler
	Dynamic Diabetes Solutions
	12091 Tretagnier Circle
	San Diego, CA 92128
	858-776-8452
	dgooler@gmail.com

Disclaimer

Dynamic Diabetes Solutions does not provide medical advice, diagnoses, or treatment for any form of diabetes or complications that may result from diabetes.

- This e-booklet contains general information about issues in the management of diabetes and complications. The information contained in this document is not medical advice, and should not be treated as such.
- You must not rely on the information in this e-booklet as an alternative to medical advice from your doctor or other professional healthcare provider.
- If you have any specific questions about any medical matter you should consult your doctor or other professional healthcare provider.
- The information in this e-booklet is for educational purposes only.

Content in E-Booklets from Dynamic Diabetes Solutions

E-booklets prepared by Dynamic Diabetes Solutions feature original writing and *aggregated information.* By aggregated information, we mean information that has been gleaned from a variety of credible web sites, and summarized as appropriate to enhance the points being made in each e-booklet.

Information referenced in this document is taken from sources that are generally readily available to the reader. Only rarely will information from a journal or other print source, not easily available to the reader, be cited. Reference to the source of previously published material is clearly identified and, insofar as possible, the URL address is provided in the reference list at the end of this booklet.

Because this e-booklet contains references to specific web sites, the authors recognize that web sites change, come, and go. All URLs identified in this e-booklet were active at the time of writing. However, it is possible that a particular web site may disappear, or be significantly altered. Therefore, advance warning is given that some web sites links may no longer be operating. Such is the nature of our very fluid Internet world.

Many people with diabetes, or those who care from them could, with enough time and effort, find many of the internet resources we cite on their own. But we find most people with diabetes have neither the time nor the inclination to conduct exhaustive searches on the web when what they need is targeted information, and they need it now!

The primary service Dynamic Diabetes Solutions provides through these e-booklets is to help readers gain access quickly and easily to information from a variety of credible sources, on a given topic.

We trust these e-booklets will be of assistance in that regard.

Complications? Why me?

Unfortunately, it happens

Some people develop health complications that can be traced back to diabetes. People adjusting to life with complications from diabetes have the added stresses of managing yet another chronic illness. This often requires the person to take additional medications, treatments, lifestyle changes, doctor's appointments and expenses, possible limitations to functioning and further changes to daily routines.

In addition to making these adjustments, transitioning to life with complications from diabetes often involves a loss and grief process, learning to cope with a new uncertainty of the future, and finding new ways to have a full and rewarding life.

Living with diabetes is difficult enough; having also to cope with a complication makes life even more challenging, and sometimes downright frightening!

Essentially, if a system or organ requires nerves, blood, or oxygen, it's fair game. Eyes, kidneys, heart, lungs, reproductive organs, skin, bones, stomach. I can't think of a system that's off-limits. It's awful to think about. So we don't. We choke it down and push it back and we don't dwell on it.

To people with diabetes, the word complication is code for "quietly life-shattering." It's a code word for failure. [2]

The American Diabetes Association (ADA) says this about diabetes and complications:

Diabetes increases your risk for many serious health problems. The good news? With the correct treatment and recommended lifestyle changes, many people with diabetes are able to prevent or delay the onset of complications. [1]

This ADA site provides information about a variety of complications that could accompany diabetes.

Preventing complications before they happen is, of course, the ideal course of action. However, life doesn't always work that way. No one deliberately sets out to get complications from their diabetes, but complications happen. And if a complication arises, the person with diabetes is compelled to deal with that complication.

In this e-booklet, we want to share five "lessons learned" for managing the emergence of a complication and diabetes. These lessons are based on scores of stories from those who are adjusting, or have had to adjust to life with complications while simultaneously dealing with their complications. Many people have made the transition successfully, and have learned some things in the process.

What are some of these complications that can be traced back to diabetes? We don't want to alarm you, but it is important to be aware of potential complications that have been demonstrated to result from or correlate positively with poorly-managed diabetes.

Possible complications of poorly-managed diabetes

First, please notice the title of this section: complications of **poorly-managed** diabetes. The words in the title have been carefully chosen. Too often, complications are linked to *diabetes,* not *poorly-managed* diabetes, and this omission can result in confusion, high levels of anxiety, and, yes, poorly-managed diabetes.

So the brief outline of complications we present to you here should be understood as being linked to poorly-managed diabetes. Let's be frank: sometimes people whose diabetes is well-managed do get complications. We know that. Still, your chances of contracting a complication to go with your diabetes are far less if your diabetes is well-managed.

So with that caveat, we describe possible complications resulting from or accompanying diabetes.

Stroke and heart attack

A stroke happens when the blood supply to part of your brain is suddenly interrupted. Then brain tissue is damaged. Most strokes happen because a blood clot blocks a blood vessel in the brain or neck. A stroke can cause movement problems, pain, numbness and problems with thinking, remembering or speaking. Some people also have emotional problems, such as depression, after a stroke. [3]

So what is the relationship between stroke and diabetes? According to the National Diabetes Information Clearinghouse:

> If you have diabetes, you are at least twice as likely as someone who does not have to have heart disease or a stroke. People with diabetes also tend to develop heart disease or have strokes at an earlier age than other people. If you are middle-aged and have type 2 diabetes, some studies suggest that your chance of having a heart attack is as high as someone without diabetes who has already had one heart attack. [4]

The web site WebMD offers this information about diabetes and stroke:

If you have diabetes, it's important to understand your increased risk of stroke. Multiple studies have shown that people with diabetes are at greater risk for stroke compared to people without diabetes -- regardless of the number of health risk factors they have. Overall, the health risk of cardiovascular disease (including stroke) is two-and-a-half times higher in men and women with diabetes compared to people without diabetes. [5]

And the Joslin Diabetes Center, a leading authority on diabetes, adds this about diabetes and heart disease:

A strong link between diabetes and heart disease is now well established. Studies from Joslin Diabetes Center several years ago showed a two- to threefold increase in the incidence of heart disease in patients with diabetes compared with those without diabetes who were being followed in the Framingham Heart Study. Women with diabetes have an even greater risk of heart disease compared with those of similar age who do not have diabetes. In fact, cardiovascular disease leading to heart attack or stroke is by far the leading cause of death in both men and women with diabetes. Another major component of cardiovascular disease is poor circulation in the legs, which contributes to a greatly increased risk of foot ulcers and amputations. [6]

There is convincing evidence of a strong relationship between diabetes and various forms of heart disease and stroke, and thus it makes sense for anyone with diabetes to be aware of this relationship, and to manage their diabetes in ways that reduce the likelihood of adding heart disease to the challenges of living with diabetes.

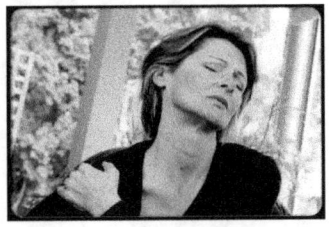

Eye complications

The American Diabetes Association provides this general statement about eye complications resulting from diabetes:

> You may have heard that diabetes causes eye problems and may lead to blindness. People with diabetes do have a higher risk of blindness than people without diabetes. But most people who have diabetes have nothing more than minor eye disorders.

> With regular checkups, you can keep minor problems minor. And if you do develop a major problem, there are treatments that often work well if you begin them right away. [7]

The ADA indicates that people with diabetes are indeed more likely to develop eye complications than people without diabetes:

- Glaucoma: People with diabetes are 40% more likely to suffer from glaucoma than people without diabetes. The longer someone has had diabetes, the more common glaucoma is. Risk also increases with age.
- Cataracts: Many people without diabetes get cataracts, but people with diabetes are 60% more likely to develop this eye condition. People with diabetes also tend to get cataracts at a younger age and have them progress faster. With cataracts, the eye's clear lens clouds, blocking light.
- Retinopathy: The longer you've had diabetes, the more likely you are to have retinopathy. Almost everyone with type 1 diabetes will eventually have nonproliferative retinopathy. And most people with type 2 diabetes will also get it. But the retinopathy that destroys vision, proliferative retinopathy, is far less common. People who keep their blood sugar levels closer to normal are less likely to have retinopathy or to have milder forms. [8]

Kidney disease

MedicineNet.com offers the following observation about diabetes and kidney disease:

Diabetes is the most common cause of kidney failure, accounting for nearly 44 percent of new cases. Even when diabetes is controlled, the disease can lead to chronic kidney disease and kidney failure. Most people with diabetes do not develop chronic kidney disease that is severe enough to progress to kidney failure. Nearly 24 million people in the United States have diabetes, and nearly 180,000 people are living with kidney failure as a result of diabetes. [9]

Medline Plus, from the National Institutes of Health, provides this summary of the relationship between diabetes and kidney disease:

If you have diabetes, your blood glucose, or blood sugar, levels are too high. Over time, this can damage your kidneys. Your kidneys clean your blood. If they are damaged, waste and fluids build up in your blood instead of leaving your body.

Kidney damage from diabetes is called diabetic nephropathy. It begins long before you have symptoms. An early sign of it is small amounts of protein in your urine. A urine test can detect it. A blood test can also help determine how well your kidneys are working.

If the damage continues, your kidneys could fail. In fact, diabetes is the most common cause of kidney failure in the United States. People with kidney failure need either dialysis or a kidney transplant.

You can slow down kidney damage or keep it from getting worse. Controlling your blood sugar and blood pressure, taking your medicines and not eating too much protein can help. [10]

There are many more potential complications resulting from or co-existing with diabetes: foot problems; ketoacidosis; gastroparesis; neuropathy. All of these are possible, *but not inevitable*. Your success at managing your diabetes will be a major factor in whether you experience any of these complications.

If you wish to learn more about the complications that are often linked to diabetes, you might want to consult any of the web sites identified below.

Diabetes and Complications
Inventory of Web Sites

Sponsor	Web site title	URL
American Diabetes Association	Complications	http://www.diabetes.org/living-with-diabetes/complications/
International Diabetes Federation	Complications of diabetes	http://www.idf.org/complications-diabetes
Mayo Clinic	Complications	http://www.mayoclinic.org/diseases-conditions/diabetes/basics/complications/con-20033091
National Library of Medicine	Long term complications of diabetes	http://www.mayoclinic.org/diseases-conditions/diabetes/basics/complications/con-20033091
JDRF	Diabetes complications	https://jdrf.org/life-with-t1d/type-1-diabetes-information/diabetes-complications/
Joslin Diabetes Center	Complications research	http://www.joslin.org/diabetes-research/diabetes-complications-research.html
Australian Diabetes Council	Diabetes complications	http://www.australiandiabetescouncil.com/about-diabetes/diabetes-complications

Wow! That's a pretty scary array of things that could happen to me. I'm not eager to have to deal with any of those complications. So, an obvious question: can these complications be prevented?

Preventing Complications? It's complicated!

I have yet to see any problem, however complicated, which when looked at in the right way did not become still more complicated.
Poul Anderson

Not surprisingly, a great deal has been written about the prevention or avoidance of complications associated with diabetes. It's not so easy for the layperson to figure out the bottom line when it comes to preventing complications. What can I do?

Here are some of the ideas "out there" about prevention of complications if you have diabetes:

The Mayo Clinic offers 10 ways to avoid diabetes complications:

1. Make a commitment to managing your diabetes.
2. Don't smoke.
3. Keep your blood pressure and cholesterol under control.
4. Schedule yearly physicals and eye examinations.
5. Keep your vaccines up to date.
6. Take care of your teeth.
7. Pay attention to your feet.
8. Consider a daily aspirin.
9. If you drink alcohol, do so responsibly.
10. Take stress seriously. [11]

The Joslin Diabetes Center offers 6 tips for avoiding complications from diabetes:

1. Take control of your blood glucose.
2. Watch your cholesterol.
3. Keep blood pressure in check.
4. Don't forget your kidneys.
5. Look out for your eyes.
6. Examine your feet. [12]

The Cleveland Clinic suggests the following basic principles for prevention of complications of diabetes:

1. Take your medications (pills and/or insulin) as prescribed by your doctor.
2. Monitor your blood sugars closely.
3. Follow a sensible diet. Do not skip meals.
4. Exercise regularly.
5. See your doctor regularly to monitor for complications. [13]

There are clearly a number of steps you can take to prevent or avoid certain complications that are often associated with diabetes, as the suggestions above outline.

If your diabetes is well-managed, complications may not be in your future. In spite of all the steps you take to keep complications out of your life by managing your diabetes, we must be realistic: complications do happen, and trying to deal with the transition to managing both your diabetes and a complication is challenging.

As promised, we want to share with you some life "lessons learned" from people who have struggled with the addition of a complication to their already complicated diabetes life. You may be disappointed (but not surprised) to learn that there are no magic formulas, no prescriptions, no single approach that is ideal when you are faced with a complication. But there are some things that, if you know about them, may make transitioning to management of a complication a little easier for you.

So here they are!

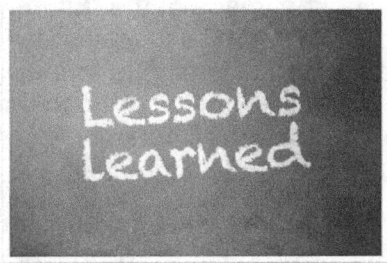

Some Lessons Learned about transitioning to a complication

1

The transition to having a complication often involves many difficult feelings.

Having diabetes, and then discovering you are about to experience a complication resulting from that diabetes, can cause a torrent of feelings, many of which are very difficult to cope with. People who are adjusting to life with complications describe varying degrees of fear, shame, guilt, anger, loss and grief, sadness, hopelessness and feeling overwhelmed. Unfortunately, many people do not discuss these feelings with anyone, including close family members and even friends who have diabetes.

Here's a brief look at some of the feeling you might well experience if you are a person with diabetes and learn you are about to have a complication.

Grief

Developing complications can present losses associated with changes of: the body's functioning, roles at home/work, relationships, identity and the image of the "future." The feelings of grief and loss that people experience in response to these changes are important to be addressed. Coming to terms with grief involves acknowledging the losses without minimizing them and working through the many feelings that go with them. The goal is to be able to move forward and not get stuck in the grief.

Grief has been defined as keen mental suffering or distress over affliction or loss; sharp sorrow; painful regret. The emotion felt by someone who has just learned he or she is on the verge of kidney failure fits the definition of grief.

Experts at the Mayo Clinic offer this observation about grief:

> When someone is newly diagnosed with a chronic disease, it's necessary to deal with grief. Any loss isn't easy and there will be periods of denial, sadness and anger. You may ask, why me? Anger can be directed towards your healthcare provider, family and friends. You may have feelings of guilt and ask yourself questions like, "Is it my fault, could I have done something different?" Are you fearful of complications? These concerns are all a part of the grieving process, which can come and go. [14]

Eric Bejarano offers this comment on grief:

> Grief needs to be understood, accepted, and dealt with, or later on it can become stronger and harder to cope with. Grieving over complications such as loss of sight, kidney dialysis, or loss of a limb creates another new form of grief where they feel guilt, denial, shock, anger, and depression all over again. [15]

What does grief feel like? Here is one description:

> When experiencing grief, it is common to:
> - Feel like you are "going crazy"
> - Have difficulty concentrating
> - Feel sad or depressed
> - Be irritable or angry (at the deceased, oneself, others, higher powers)
> - Feel frustrated or misunderstood
> - Experience anxiety, nervousness, or fearfulness
> - Feel like you want to "escape"
> - Experience guilt or remorse
> - Be ambivalent
> - Feel numb
> - Lack energy and motivation [16]

Anger

Anger, an emotion with which we are all familiar, is one of the feelings you may have when you learn of a complication. The American Diabetes Association argues that diabetes and anger often go together:

> Diabetes is the perfect breeding ground for anger. Anger can start at diagnosis with the question, "Why me?" You may dwell on how unfair diabetes is: "I'm so angry at this disease! I don't want to treat it. I don't want to control it. I hate it!"

> One reason diabetes and anger so often go hand in hand is that diabetes can make you feel threatened. Life with diabetes can seem full of dangers - insulin reactions or complications. When you fear these threats, anger often surges to your defense.

> While it's true that out-of-control anger can cause more harm than good, that's only part of the story. Anger can also help you assert and protect yourself. You can learn to use your anger. You can even put it to work for better diabetes care. [17]

Anger is a normal reaction to being diagnosed with diabetes; it is no less normal to feel anger toward the complication that has been added to your life.

We've probably all learned at various points in our lives that anger is not always a bad thing. Problems arise when we fail to get beyond the anger:

> It's ok to get angry. Scream at your diabetes; tell it how much you hate it, how much you wish it would go away. But don't let the anger take you over. It takes a lot of energy to be angry, and you're going to need that energy to manage your disease.

This anger will probably always be with you in one form or another, such as frustration with your treatment program, restrictions on what you can eat, the constant need to exercise, the drugs you have to take. When that occurs, take a few minutes to feel and acknowledge that anger; then remind yourself of the possible alternatives—blindness, kidney failure and dialysis, heart disease, strokes, amputations, and an earlier death—and continue the program that will stop these complications from occurring. [18]

Add a complication on top of your diabetes? How could you not be angry? Expect the anger, let it flow for a time, but don't let it hurt you or someone else. And especially, don't let anger prevent you from managing your diabetes and your complication.

Despair

You may also experience feelings of despair about your new complication, perhaps having a sense that everything is wrong and nothing will turn out well.

Despair is unpleasant and may evolve into its more serious form, depression. Here's one account of despair:

Oh, that painful word despair. Despair brings me misery and makes me feel hopeless. Despair makes me feel anguish, gloom, and despondent to my daily activities. Sometimes I lose hope, or else give up hope. Sometimes I cannot see the light, while other times I feel dejection taking me over. What can I do? What is wrong? Am I going crazy?

No, you are not going crazy. If that were the case millions of other, people would be standing on the crazy line as well. Sometimes you may do foolish things. Sometimes you may act idiotic; however, you are not crazy. Everyday, someone just like you feels the same way. Therefore, do not think you are alone. [19]

Helplessness

When diagnosed with a complication, on top of your diabetes, you may feel overwhelmed, helpless, and hopeless. Practically, you may feel powerless or unable to act independently.

Initial feelings of helplessness can evolve into something called *learned helplessness*. When people feel that they have no control over their situation (such as having a complication of some kind associated with diabetes), they may also begin to behave in a helpless manner. This inaction can lead people to overlook opportunities for relief or change. [20]

One of the most common manifestations of a feeling of helplessness and hopelessness is depression. Depression will be discussed later in this e-booklet.

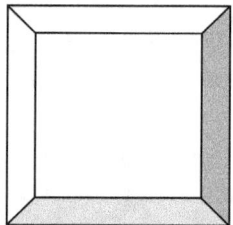

Grief; anger; despair; helplessness: These are some of the possible tough feelings you will have as you learn you have a complication related to your diabetes. Knowing you may get these feelings doesn't solve the underlying issues, of course, but knowing may make it easier for you to recognize and cope with the tough feelings.

If or when these feelings happen to you, know that you are not losing your mind, you are not weak, you have not failed. And, you are not alone!

2 | Be aware of your own self-criticism about having complications.

Why am I getting this complication? Is it something I did, or didn't do?

People with diabetes + complications often blame themselves for both the diabetes and the complication, suffer from feeling of self-blame, and end up ashamed of themselves. The consequences of these feelings of shame and blame can be detrimental to self-management of the new complication and the diabetes. If you are a person with diabetes, and you've learned you are "acquiring" a complication, you may find yourself deeply critical of your own behavior; you may feel culpable for somehow inviting the complication.

A study called the United Kingdom Prospective Diabetes Study (UKPDS) has stimulated a number of publications, including one that bears directly on self-criticism about having complications pertaining to diabetes. This article, titled *Diabetes through the Life Span: Psychological Ramifications for Patients and Professionals*, provides important insight into the issue of self-criticism. Following are several brief segments from the paper:

> For some people, the reaction to a new diagnosis taps hidden resources, resiliency, even a new-found spirituality. For others, the emotional pain is hard to integrate. Until grief for the various losses is confronted, it may be too painful for patients to face the problem of management with full awareness.

> An individual's adaptation to diabetes requires emotional awareness and skills to meet daily challenges from existing complications, stress, dietary choices, exercising, blood testing, taking medications, and making decisions. How effectively these challenges are met will be influenced by the individual's personality dynamics, unfinished business in dealing with past losses, level of family function, family life cycle stage, gender, and cultural perspective. [21]

Can diabetes effect self-esteem? The American Diabetes Association posted this answer to the question:

>Unfortunately, diabetes can gnaw away at your sense of self-worth. Some people with diabetes blame themselves for having the illness or its complications. Sometimes, people think less of themselves because they feel different. This can happen whether you are a child, a teenager, or an adult. Some people even wonder if they are being punished when they get diabetes. [22]

Or a complication.

There are people who blame themselves for complications. Check out what this person said:

>How many of us out there blame ourselves for any diabetic complications they have? how many do not?
>
>I can't help blaming myself even though I know the odds were stacked against me in some ways, I was in denial over my diabetes for many years (getting diagnosed as a teenager didn't help, I was far too young to take on the responsibility and once I had experienced a period of time 'getting away with it' it got harder and harder to pick that responsibility up as the years went by). However I also had an eating disorder which pre dated the diabetes and felt totally out of control where food was concerned. This lead to under injecting (a form of diabulimia I suppose) which although I was perfectly aware was very wrong, I felt powerless to stop.
>This lead to retinopathy, which ironically when my blood sugars were at their lowest (when pregnant) combined with pregnancy hormones, lead to the need for laser treatment.

I do feel guilty, although I also feel the medical profession did not do enough to help me either with the eating disorder or with the diabetes (e.g., when first put on insulin was told to take set amounts of fast acting, not to carb count or match to meals) and still I feel that I am on my own in many ways as I don't have much faith in the medical profession to understand how hard it can be to manage this condition. [23]

As suggested above, people with diabetes who develop complications are critical of themselves for developing the complication. These individuals feel blame for their condition, and often also feel shame as a result. Shame and blame are sometimes referred to as *stigma*. Stigma has been defined as "a set of negative and often unfair beliefs that a society or group of people have about something." [24]. The shame and blame feelings that accompany diagnosis of a complication are a stigma often assigned to a person by him or herself.

Social stigma is defined as a strong social disapproval of characteristics or beliefs seen as being against the cultural norms. What is stigmatized varies depending on the social and political contexts employed by society. People get stigmatized due to factors like mental illness, physical disabilities and diseases. [25]

A recent research study conducted by Browne et al [26] sought to explore the social experiences of Australian adults living with type 2 diabetes mellitus (T2DM), with a particular focus on the perception and experience of diabetes-related stigma. While the study was about diabetes, not complications, the results are applicable to the feeling of shame and blame about getting complications:

A total of 21 (84%) participants indicated that they believed T2DM was stigmatised, or reported evidence of stigmatisation. Specific themes about the experience of stigma were feeling blamed by others for causing their own condition, being subject to negative stereotyping, being discriminated against or having restricted opportunities in life. Other themes focused on sources of stigma, which included the media, healthcare professionals, friends, family and colleagues. Themes relating to the consequences of this stigma were also evident, including participants' unwillingness to disclose their condition to others and psychological distress.

In a blog, Martha Zimmer made a strong point about the potential dangers of shame:

Shame will never help anyone to change. Books have been written by psychologists who observe the damage. Teachers who use shame on their students get fired when they are caught.

Shame gives the message "I am a bad person." There is no cure for that, if you believe it. And it is a small step from guilt to shame for many. [27]

It's time to stop the shame/blame talk!

David Kendall, M.D., is the chief scientific and medical officer of the American Diabetes Association. He says:

No one is to blame for their diabetes. We certainly cannot control the genes we inherit. And while certain environmental and behavior "triggers" have been identified, managing those risk factors can be challenging.

We do know that diabetes can be effectively managed and that by working to control blood glucose levels, people with diabetes can reduce their risk of developing complications. For people with type 2 diabetes, moderate weight loss can be helpful; for everyone with diabetes, eating a healthy diet, increasing physical activity, and using their medications as prescribed are all helpful in the management of this disease. [28]

Rita Rubin, well known in the diabetes community, in an article titled "Diabetes shame plus denial a risky combo," relayed the following:

Few chronic diseases carry more stigma than Type 2 diabetes. While patients with heart disease or cancer are often showered with sympathy, people with Type 2 diabetes are criticized for being fat, lazy or junk food junkies.

Even diabetics themselves can have a blame-the-victim feeling, says Theresa Garnero, a diabetes nurse educator at the California Pacific Medical Center in San Francisco.

The problem is, shame plus denial, especially with loved ones or medical professionals, can be a risky combination when it comes to managing diabetes, experts warn. People who hide their condition may not be as careful about monitoring their blood sugar or eating healthfully. [29]

We all can do better at managing our diabetes, but we put ourselves in some jeopardy if we are overly self-critical, and accept shame and blame, especially concerning complications.

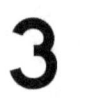 **3** You are not imagining it: There are good reasons why you feel you are struggling with your diabetes, and why you wonder if you can cope with a complication.

Diabetes management is a big job. Life with complications can make the job even bigger. People struggle with diabetes for many different reasons, and often feel people around them do not understand how complicated life is with diabetes. Obstacles to good management on a daily basis can stack up so high that you sometimes can't see the benefits of good management because the challenges overwhelm you. Add a complication: it becomes even more difficult to see the benefits of giving so much effort to managing your diabetes. Why bother?

> Diabetes is a chronic disease and it doesn't go away. Once diagnosed, the patient and health care team navigate changes in diet, exercise, weight management, and medication. With the news of diabetes, most patients report more office visits and more lab tests. Patients are asked to test blood sugar at home and make follow-up appointments if the numbers are not in an expected range. Diabetes sets into motion a series of changes that impact our daily routine and often affects everyone in your family in some way. Is it any wonder that everyone with diabetes faces struggles with 'following the rules' at some points in their journey with the disease? [30]

What are these obstacles to good diabetes management, and to the effective management of a complication? There are many:

- Lack of knowledge or skill ("I don't understand carbohydrate counting")
  - Harmful health beliefs ("Diabetes is a death sentence"; "Starting insulin means I have failed")
  - Patient/Doctor communication problems ("I can't tell my doctor what I am really doing")

- Unachievable goals ("I need to lose 30 pounds before my next visit"; "My doctor wants my A1C at 6% and I don't know why")
- Treatment side effects/interactions ("My cholesterol medication gave me muscle pain", "My antidepressant makes my blood pressure higher")
- Poor social support or diabetes police ("I don't have anyone in my life who supports my diabetes efforts"; "My wife is constantly scolding me for what I eat")
- Ineffective coping skills ("I binge eat when I am stressed")
- Environmental barriers ("I don't have health insurance and strips are expensive")
- Elements of diabetes that get in the way ("I finally have my A1C down and now I am having scary hypoglycemia"; "Exercise and eating carefully must have stopped working for me because now I am told I need more medication")
- Other illnesses/complications ("My gastro paresis makes it really hard to manage my blood sugars after I eat."; "The diet recommended for my kidney disease makes me feel even more limited.")
- Depression ("Depression makes it nearly impossible for me to care about checking my blood sugars and watching my diet. Sometimes, I don't even care about getting out of bed.")

Given all these obstacles to achieving good management of your diabetes, and given the possibility of a looming complication, what can you do?

A good place to start is to know in some detail what obstacles are getting in your way of good management, and then work with your diabetes healthcare professional to tackle these obstacles, one at a time. **You can't overcome all the barriers at once; you will become frustrated if you try**. But solving one obstacle at a time makes the task manageable, and you can feel some success. Understanding and planning for the obstacles to your efforts to manage diabetes can help you succeed in areas where you may have struggled in the past. And overcoming, or at least reducing, these barriers will make it more likely you can deal effectively with a complication.

4   There will be Ups And Downs In your diabetes management with a complication

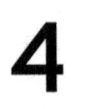

You know how challenging it is, on a daily basis, to manage your diabetes. If you learn you may be acquiring a complication, or if you've already been diagnosed with a complication and have begun to treat the complication, you are likely to find it even more challenging to achieve a satisfactory level of diabetes management.

Why? The simple answer is: priorities.

You only have so much time, so much effort, and so much knowledge. When you get a complication, some of that time, effort, and knowledge must necessarily be diverted to deal with the new complication, thus reducing the amount of time and effort available to deal with your diabetes.

There is no magic formula about priorities when it comes to managing both your diabetes and a complication. There are, however, four priorities that seem of importance no matter your personal situation.

Priority #1: Do not fail to take your prescribed medications.

Even if you are feeling overwhelmed by the challenges of managing multiple chronic illnesses, it is vital that you not stop taking medications that have been prescribed for your diabetes. Why?

A reader posed this question: What are the side effects of not taking diabetes medication? Answer?
> Moodiness, swelling, death, weight gain, dysfunctional thinking, and memory loss. [31]

Clearly not good! A physician offered his perspective on issues associated with failing to take prescribed medication:

The extent of the problem of "primary medication non-adherence" (not filling the initial prescription for a new drug) became much clearer with the publication of a study in the April 2010 issue of the Journal of General Internal Medicine that found that a whopping 28% of new prescriptions were never filled.

While anyone who has ever tried to complete a full course of antibiotics can understand how easy it is to skip, cut down or forget one's medications altogether, bringing the topic up in the exam room feels more like a confession or inquisition than a rational discussion. Few of us want to talk about medication non-adherence, much less admit to it.

Fair enough. But there are plenty of good reasons to change this mindset. Prescriptions that aren't filled can't do any good, but they can easily do harm: for example, in the diabetic patient who is hospitalized for an infection and given his "regular" insulin dose, only to become comatose from low blood sugar because he never actually took that dose (which his puzzled physician kept increasing) in real life. [32]

Results of a 2006 study revealed that:

...people who did not adhere to their drug regimens had a 58% greater chance of ending up in the hospital and an 81% greater chance of dying than those who did adhere, even when other factors that may have contributed to these outcomes were accounted for... the takeaway message from these studies seems clear (take your medicine as directed!).

The researchers understand that people with diabetes or heart disease who do not take their medicines regularly are not the only ones at fault—poor communication between health-care professionals and patients also contributes to nonadherence. They urge health-care professionals to assess whether or not people are taking their medicines during routine appointments. Other researchers suggest additional interventions such as electronic reminders for doctors, automated voice messages for people using drug therapy, and outreach from pharmacy staff. [33]

Priority #2: Agree on a treatment plan with your physician and health care team, and stick with it.

A study of one hundred twenty-seven pairs of patients and their primary care physicians in two health systems were surveyed about their top 3 diabetes treatment goals (desired outcomes) and strategies to meet those goals. The results?

…patients with more education, greater belief in the efficacy of their diabetes treatment, and who shared in treatment decision making with their providers were more likely to agree with their providers on treatment goals or strategies. Similarly, physician reports of having discussed more content areas of diabetes self-care were associated with greater agreement on treatment strategies. *In turn, greater agreement on treatment goals and strategies was associated both with higher patient diabetes care self-efficacy and assessments of their diabetes self-management.* (Italics added) [34]

Collaboration with your health care team thus seems critical to effective self-management of diabetes, especially in light of complications. Adding to this point is the following:

In addition to the importance of clear physician provision of information, collaborative physician styles have been found to result in higher patient satisfaction and adherence to treatment plans, 16 and patient–provider agreement on treatment goals and strategies has been associated with higher levels of chronic disease self-efficacy and self-management. 17 In such collaborative interactions, both patient and physician share responsibility for identifying and solving problems, for setting and achieving realistic goals, for monitoring progress, and for developing and adapting treatment strategies as necessary. [35]

Priority #3: Engage your family and friends in helping you manage your diabetes while coping with a complication.

The crucial role a loved one can play in the life of a person with diabetes who is also dealing with, or about to deal with, a complication, cannot be overstated. Just how a family member or friend of a person with diabetes can provide needed support was described nicely in an article on the web site dlife:

> As a caregiver, helping your loved one to avoid debilitating and costly complications starts by encouraging or even helping them to manage their diabetes effectively. A proper diet, exercise, and regular medical visits are your best defense against this disease.
>
> Complications are a scary subject. Never treat a complication as "punishment" for poor diabetes care. They can happen even to those who try their hardest to attain good diabetes control. Even if a complication is truly the result of poor diabetes care, reminding your loved one of that fact does nothing to help the situation or your relationship.

If your loved one has already developed some complications related to their diabetes, work with them to prevent further damage by managing blood sugars to the best of their ability and treating the complication appropriately. To find out more about diabetes-related complications and how to support the person in your life with diabetes, learn more about how diabetes impacts the different organ systems of the body. [36]

So if you see the value in getting family and friends involved in your self-management of diabetes and possible complications, how do you go about achieving that involvement? Cox Health offers some suggestions:

- Ask them to attend diabetes education classes and diabetes support groups with you. This will help them understand what you need to do to manage your diabetes and in many cases family members find that they are helped by adopting many of the behavioral changes themselves.
- Provide your family with information and encourage them to participate in activities like those sponsored by the American Diabetes Association and the Juvenile Diabetes Research Foundation.
- Practice skills at home with your family and discuss the treatment for low blood sugar so family and friends can understand what you go through and how to help you if needed.
- Share with your support group your meal and medication schedule. Tell them how you plan to handle any schedule changes so they're prepared in the event of complications.
- Encourage any family member who is having trouble coping with your having diabetes to seek counseling to discuss his or her feelings and/or anxieties.

- Let others know how they can help you: "It really helps me when I see you order healthy foods off the menu first." Let them know how you feel about them eating sweet foods and desserts in front of you. Some people find it difficult to not eat what everyone else has; others don't mind at all when their friends have sweet foods. Clear the air with your friends, and cast off everyone's uncertainty about what to do.
- Ask a family member or friend to join you in an exercise or weight control program. [37]

Priority #4: Don't be critical of yourself if you occasionally "fail" in your diabetes self-management when also dealing with a complication.

You are a person with diabetes. By definition, you are not perfect. Your diabetes management will not be perfect. When faced with a coming complication, your diabetes management is likely to be even less perfect than before the complication. Please, do not beat yourself up when things are not as perfect as you would like.

Looking at diabetes control in an oversimplified, all-or-nothing way leaves perfectionists with only two possible outcomes. Either they succeed in achieving their goals, or they fail. For a perfectionist, anything short of complete success can feel like a failure. Almost is not usually good enough. If the perfectionist is the clinician, almost may not be good enough for them, either. Some patients will get so frustrated with their inability to achieve perfect control that they will give up altogether. This is when perfectionism can be a problem. [38]

Here are two additional thoughts to consider if you are concerned about "failing" at your diabetes management while dealing with a new complication:

People frequently discuss diabetes-related behavior in terms that position themselves or others as disobedient children, or as wicked or foolish adults. These references occur alongside appraisals of the physical and social complexity of "compliance" with diabetic regimes and in some instances the difficulty of achieving effective control over blood sugar levels. Efforts to protect themselves from the stigmatizing potential of diabetes may inadvertently undermine the agency of people who are already coping with a demanding discipline and a potentially disabling or life-threatening disease. [39]

With diabetes, we have even more reasons to feel less-than-perfect. That diet you promised to start. That exercise plan you committed to. The blood sugar results you're supposed to record. If you are human, you've made commitments in all sincerity and you've "failed" at them, and felt pretty bad about it. Or, if you are the parent of someone with diabetes, undoubtedly you have not been able to maintain perfect blood sugars and perfectly "normal" life for and with your child. Spiraling negatively with guilt, shame and self-blame gives us higher stress hormones, limits our relationships, and negatively affects our lives. [40]

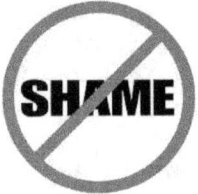 

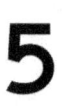 **5** **Be very aware of early signs of depression, and seek treatment as soon as you can.**

People with diabetes are more likely to develop depression than many other people, and those who have multiple complications from diabetes are at greatest risk. A study by Anderson concluded: "The presence of diabetes doubles the odds of comorbid depression." [41]

With depression, diabetes can become harder to handle and blood sugars are likely to rise. When diabetes is out of control, this can make it even harder to escape depression. It becomes a vicious cycle.

The linkage between diabetes and depression has been explicated in numerous research studies. The topic is much larger than can be explored in any detail in this e-booklet. Because the link between diabetes and depression is so strong, and because having a complication will only escalate the diabetes-depression link, it may be useful to review a very small sample of the literature on the topic.

The National Institute of Mental Health posed the question: How are depression and diabetes linked?

> Studies show that depression and diabetes may be linked, but scientists do not yet know whether depression increases the risk of diabetes or diabetes increases the risk of depression. Current research suggests that both cases are possible.
> In addition to possibly increasing your risk for depression, diabetes may make symptoms of depression worse. The stress of managing diabetes every day and the effects of diabetes on the brain may contribute to depression. In the United States, people with diabetes are twice as likely as the average person to have depression.

At the same time, some symptoms of depression may reduce overall physical and mental health, not only increasing your risk for diabetes but making diabetes symptoms worse. For example, overeating may cause weight gain, a major risk factor for diabetes. Fatigue or feelings of worthlessness may cause you to ignore a special diet or medication plan needed to control your diabetes, worsening your diabetes symptoms. Studies have shown that people with diabetes and depression have more severe diabetes symptoms than people who have diabetes alone. [42]

WebMD reported:

Depression increased the risk for diabetes, and diabetes increased the risk for depression, the study shows. Specifically, women who were depressed were 17% more likely to develop diabetes even after the researchers adjusted for other risk factors such as weight and lack of regular exercise.
Those women who were taking antidepressants were 25% more likely to develop diabetes than their counterparts who were not depressed, the study shows.

Women with diabetes were 29% more likely to develop depression after taking into account other depression risk factors, and those women who took insulin for their diabetes were 53% more likely to develop depression during the 10-year study. [43]

The Mayo Clinic offered this about the diabetes-depression connection:

If you have diabetes, you have an increased risk of developing depression. And if you have depression, you have a greater chance of developing type 2 diabetes. The good news is that diabetes and depression can be treated together. And effectively managing one can have a positive outcome on the other.

Though the relationship between diabetes and depression isn't fully understood:

- The rigors of managing diabetes can be stressful and lead to symptoms of depression.
- Diabetes can cause complications and health problems that may worsen symptoms of depression.
- Depression can lead to poor lifestyle decisions, such as unhealthy eating, less exercise, smoking and weight gain — all of which are risk factors for diabetes.
- Depression affects your ability to perform tasks, communicate and think clearly. This can interfere with your ability to successfully manage

The prevalence of depression is approximately twice as high in people with diabetes as it is in the general population. The good news is that there are effective treatments to help you to break free from depression. In turn, this can free up your energy to become more active in your diabetes care. [44]

Summary

You have diabetes, and now you learn you have an impending complication resulting from or related to your diabetes. You now have to start thinking about how you will manage both your diabetes and this new complication.

In this e-booklet, we've said that there are five things you might expect to happen during the period following the diagnosis of a complication:

1. **The transition to having a complication often involves many difficult feelings.** If you know these feelings may be coming, you may be able to acknowledge the feelings and deal with them better than if the feelings catch you by surprise.
2. **Be aware of your own self-criticism about having complications.** You may have a tendency to blame yourself for your complication, and feel some shame about it.
3. **You are not imagining it: There are good reasons why you feel you are struggling with your diabetes, and why you wonder if you can cope with a complication.** You may start to think this shouldn't be so difficult, that you are a failure if you find it hard to cope with diabetes and a complication. You're not a failure: this management is very hard work.
4. **There will be Ups And Downs In your diabetes management with a complication.** Don't demand perfection of yourself: it isn't going to happen! You do the best you can.
5. **Be very aware of early signs of depression, and seek treatment as soon as you can.** Depression is serious business. Act on it!

Complications from your diabetes are very scary things. We all fear complications. But if one comes along, you can deal with it. Knowing what you are up against is a first step in exercising positive responses to complications. You can do it!

References

1   Complications. American Diabetes Association Web site.
         Retrieved January 20, 2014. http://www.diabetes.org/living-
         with-diabetes/complications/

2.   Complication. A blog post from May 29, 2013. *Sweetly voiced*
         blog. Retrieved January 20, 2014.
         http://www.sweetlyvoiced.com/2013/05/complication.html

3   Stroke. American Diabetes Association Web site. Retrieved
         January 20, 2014. http://www.diabetes.org/living-with-
         diabetes/complications/stroke.html

4   Diabetes, heart disease, and stroke. National Diabetes
         Information Clearinghouse web site. Retrieved January 20, 2014.
         http://diabetes.niddk.nih.gov/dm/pubs/stroke/DM_Heart_Strok
         e_508.pdf

5   Stroke and diabetes. WebMD web site. Retrieved January 20,
         2014. http://www.webmd.com/diabetes/guide/diabetes-stroke

6   Diabetes and Heart Disease — An Intimate Connection. Joslin
         Diabetes Center web site. Retrieved January 20, 2014.
         http://www.joslin.org/info/diabetes_and_heart_disease_an_int
         imate_connection.html

7   Eye complications. American Diabetes Association. Retrieved
         January 28, 2014, at: http://www.diabetes.org/living-with-
         diabetes/complications/eye-complications/

8   Eye complications. American Diabetes Association. Retrieved
         January 28, 2014, at: http://www.diabetes.org/living-with-
         diabetes/complications/eye-complications/

9   Diabetes and kidney disease. MedicineNet.com. Retrieved on
         January 28, 2014, at:
         http://www.medicinenet.com/diabetes_and_kidney_disease/pa
         ge2.htm

10   Diabetic kidney problems. Medline Plus. National Library of
         Medicine, National Institutes of Health. Retrieved on January 28,
         2014, at:
         http://www.nlm.nih.gov/medlineplus/diabetickidneyproblems.
         html

11   Diabetes care: 10 ways to avoid diabetes complications. The
         Mayo Clinic. Retrieved on January 28, 2014, at:
         http://www.mayoclinic.org/diseases-conditions/diabetes/in-
         depth/diabetes-management/ART-20045803?pg=1

12   6 tips for avoiding complications from diabetes. Joslin Diabetes
         Center. Retrieved on January 28, 2014, at:
         http://www.joslin.org/info/6_tips_for_avoiding_complications_
         from_diabetes.html

13   Preventing diabetes complications. Cleveland Clinic web site.
         Retrieved on March 26, 2014, at:

http://my.clevelandclinic.org/disorders/diabetes_mellitus/hic_preventing_the_complications_of_diabetes.aspx

14   Grief is a natural reaction to diabetes diagnosis. Living with diabetes blog. Mayo Clinic. Retrieved on January 28, 2014 at: http://www.mayoclinic.org/diseases-conditions/diabetes/expert-blog/diabetes-diagnosis/BGP-20056544

15   Eric Bejarano. Diabetes: Unmasking Its Hidden Toll. Oandp.com. Retrieved on January 28, 2014 at: http://www.oandp.com/articles/2006-03_04.asp

16   Grief and loss. University of Texas. Retrieved on March 27, 2014, at: http://cmhc.utexas.edu/griefloss.html

17   Anger. American Diabetes Association. Retrieved on January 28, 2014, at: http://www.diabetes.org/living-with-diabetes/complications/mental-health/anger.html

18   Coping with a diabetes diagnosis. The Complete Idiot's Guide to Diabetes. Retrieved on January 28, 2014, at: http://idiotsguides.com/static/quickguides/healthbeautydiet/coping-with-a-diabetes-diagnosis.html

19   How to Manage Despair and Conquer Depression. Retrieved on March 27, 2014, at: http://depression.readabout.net/Despair-in-How-to-Manage-and-Conquer-Depression.html

20   (n.d.). Retrieved from http://www.merriam-webster.com/dictionary/stigma

21   Rapaport, W., Cohen, R., and Riddle, M. (2000). Diabetes Through the Life Span: Psychological Ramifications for Patients and Professionals. Diabetes Spectrum, Vol. 13, #4, p. 201. Retrieved January 6, 2014, at: http://journal.diabetes.org/diabetesspectrum/00v13n4/page201.asp

22   Can diabetes affect self-esteem? American Diabetes Association. Retrieved on January 28, 2014, at: http://www.sharecare.com/health/living-with-diabetes/relationship-self-esteem-diabetes

23   If you have complications - do you blame yourself? Diabetes.co.uk. Retrieved on January 28, 2014, at: http://www.diabetes.co.uk/forum/threads/if-you-have-complications-do-you-blame-yourself.21002/

24   (n.d.). Retrieved from http://www.merriam-webster.com/dictionary/stigma

25   Definition of social stigma. (n.d.). Retrieved from: http://www.ask.com/question/definition-of-social-stigma

26   Browne, J. et al (2013). 'I call it the blame and shame disease': a qualitative study about perceptions of social stigma surrounding type 2 diabetes. BMJ Open, Vol. 3. Retrieved on March 27, 2014, at: http://bmjopen.bmj.com/content/3/11/e003384.full

27   Type 2 diabetic guilt, blaming, and shaming. A diabetic life.
      Retrieved on March 27, 2014, at: http://www.a-diabetic-
      life.com/type-2-diabetic-guilt.html

28   With diabetes, don't focus on blame. David Kendall, M.D.
      Retrieved on January 28, 2014, at:
      http://thechart.blogs.cnn.com/2011/04/15/with-diabetes-dont-
      focus-on-blame/

29   Rita Rubin. Diabetes shame plus denial a risky combo. Today
      Health. Retrieved on January 29, 2014 at:
      http://www.today.com/id/45137643/ns/today-
      today_health/t/diabetes-shame-plus-denial-risky-combo/

30   Julie Paff. Struggles and Silver Linings with Diabetes. Good
      Health. Retrieved on January 29, 2014, at:
      http://www.goodhealth.com/articles/2013/04/16/struggles_and
      _silver_linings_with_diabetes

31   What are the side effects of not taking diabetes medication?
      Retrieved on January 29, 2014, at:
      http://wiki.answers.com/Q/What_are_the_side_effects_not_tak
      ing_diabetes_medication

32   When patients don't take their prescription drugs. KevinMD.
      Retrieved on February 29, 2014, at:
      http://www.kevinmd.com/blog/2010/06/patients-prescription-
      drugs.html

33   Not Taking Prescribed Drugs Linked with Death in People with
      Diabetes. Diabetes self-management blog. Retrieved on January
      29, 2014, at:
      http://www.diabetesselfmanagement.com/Blog/Tara-
      Dairman/not_taking_prescribed_drugs_linked_with_death_in_
      people_with_diabetes/

34   When Do Patients and Their Physicians Agree on Diabetes
      Treatment Goals and Strategies, and What Difference Does It
      Make? Retrieved on January 29, 2014, at:
      http://www.ncbi.nlm.nih.gov/pmc/articles/PMC1494939/

35   Michele Heisler. Actively Engaging Patients in Treatment Decision
      Making and Monitoring as a Strategy to Improve Hypertension
      Outcomes in Diabetes Mellitus. Retrieved on January 29, 2014,
      at: http://circ.ahajournals.org/content/117/11/1355.full

36   Complications and other risks. Dlife. Retrieved on January 29,
      2014, at: http://www.dlife.com/diabetes/lifestyle/diabetes-
      caregivers/caregiver_complications_and_risks

37   How can I get friends and family involved in my care? CoxHealth.
      Retrieved on January 29, 2014, at:
      http://www.coxhealth.com/body.cfm?id=3879#friendsfamily

38   Monica Ramirez Basco. Perfectionism and Diabetes Care.
      Diabetes Spectrum

Volume 11 Number 1, 1998, Pages 43-48. Retrieved on January 29, 2014, at:
http://journal.diabetes.org/diabetesspectrum/98v11n1/pg43.htm

39   Controlling diabetes, controlling diabetics: moral language in the management of diabetes type 2. Social Science & Medicine Volume 58, Issue 11, June 2004, Pages 2371–2382. Retrieved on January 29, 2014 at:
http://www.sciencedirect.com/science/article/pii/S0277953603004659

40   Let self-compassion guide how you live with your diabetes. Transforming Diabetes. Retrieved on January 29, 2014, at:
http://transformingdiabetes.com/tag/self-compassion/

41   Anderson, R.J, et al. The Prevalence of Comorbid Depression in Adults with Diabetes
A meta-analysis. Retrieved on January 29, 2014, at:
http://care.diabetesjournals.org/content/24/6/1069.full

42   Depression and diabetes. National Institute of Mental Health. Retrieved on January 29, 2014, at:
http://www.nimh.nih.gov/health/publications/depression-and-diabetes/index.shtml

43   New Links Seen Between Depression and Diabetes. WebMD. Retrieved on January 29, 2014, at:
http://www.webmd.com/depression/news/20101122/new-links-seen-between-depression-and-diabetes

44   What's the connection between diabetes and depression? Retrieved on March 29, 2014, at:
http://www.mayoclinic.org/diseases-conditions/diabetes/expert-answers/diabetes-and-depression/faq-20057904